Praise for *The Moon Reminded Me*

"Ellen O'Brian invites us into her soul, the space where poetry is born. Here human individuality engages with a wider Self. In this contemplative space words point to the concrete realities that unveil another Reality. Accept this invitation—this is good company to be in."
—KABIR HELMINSKI, translator of Rumi, author of *Living Presence*

"These glimpses into the spacious love of the Divine are testaments to Ellen's awakening and invitations to your own. Savor this book."
—Rabbi Rami Shapiro, author of *Accidental Grace*

"These poems illuminate the soul, delicately, lightly, with measured emotion. Ellen Grace O'Brian manages to express spiritual practice as life, beyond doctrine, and straight to the heart. 'Be a jagged edge/falling in love/one salty kiss/at a time.'"
—NORMAN FISCHER, poet and Zen Buddhist priest, author of *What Is Zen?: Plain Talk for a Beginner's Mind*

"In *The Moon Reminded Me*, Yogacharya Ellen Grace O'Brian presents a rare combination of deep yogic vision and intricate poetic skill, awakening us to our inner journey of Self-realization."
—DR. DAVID FRAWLEY D.LITT., author of *Vedic Yoga: The Path of the Rishi*

"In her book, *The Moon Reminded Me*, Yogacharya Ellen Grace O'Brian has so gracefully shared her life's journey, depth of her insight and devotion in a most meaningful language of poetry. Highly recommended."
—NAHID ANGHA, Sufi scholar, executive editor of *Sufism Journal*

"In her savory, contemplative verse, Yogacharya O'Brian crosses and penetrates the boundaries of tradition. Like Whitman, she illuminates the transcendent in the immanent. Like Leonard Cohen, she points to the light that enters the cracks in everything, even despair. Like the Zen poets, she evokes the sublime in the ordinary. Like the psalmists and bhaktas, she sings out in praise and cries out with longing for God, which is, in itself, a divine connection."
—PHILIP GOL̲ ̲ ̲ ̲ ̲ ̲ of *American Veda: How In*

D1429772

THE
MOON
REMINDED ME

THE
MOON
REMINDED ME

ELLEN GRACE O'BRIAN
FOREWORD BY MIRABAI STARR

HOMEBOUND PUBLICATIONS
Ensuring the mainstream isn't the only stream

HOMEBOUND PUBLICATIONS
Ensuring the mainstream isn't the only stream.

Copyright © 2017 by Ellen Grace O'Brian
All Rights Reserved
Printed in the United States of America
as well as the United Kingdom and Australia.

First Edition Trade Paperback
Paperback ISBN 978-1-938846-99-1

Front Cover Image © Elina Li | Shutterstock.com
Cover and Interior Designed by Leslie M. Browning

www.homeboundpublications.com

10 9 8 7 6 5 4 3 2 1

Homebound Publications greatly values the natural environment and invests in environmental conservation. Our books are printed on paper with chain of custody certification from the Forest Stewardship Council, Sustainable Forestry Initiative, and the Program for the Endorsement of Forest Certification. In addition, each year Homebound Publications donates 1% of our net profit to a humanitarian or ecological charity.

For Amarnāth

CONTENTS

FOREWORD
A NOTE FROM MIRABAI STARR

When I was a teenager, I fell in love with Krishna. While my peers were forming rock bands and sharing bottles of sweet wine, I was composing love poems to the god of love and chanting myself into a trance. My first boyfriend had been killed in an accident right around the time I was cast in the leading role of Mirabai, the sixteenth century Indian saint, in a school musical and the name stuck. Grief for my human love and longing for God collided and have been intermingled ever since.

Yogacharya Ellen Grace O'Brian gets the connection between the holy fire of devotion and the blessed waters of ordinary life. In this exquisite collection of poems, she freely dances between the sublime discontent of a soul suffering from the illusion of separation from its beloved source, what it's like to navigate the deaths of three close friends, and still remain fully awake in the world. She celebrates the way the branches of an apple tree reach starkly for the sky in winter and she makes a place for the Divine Mother at the table of her soul. In one breath she rushes like a thirsty deer to the waters of prayer and in the next she tells a little tale about four glass bowls and a monk.

The poet is not limited to a single tradition, and she invites us to join her at the inter-spiritual party. *I wonder* (Ellen wonders in "Svadharma"): / *are the frogs saying* Allah! Allah! / *Or* Rama, Rama, Rama? / *Perhaps it's* Jesus! Jesus! And she concludes in "One Name" that all creation praises the Holy in its own special voice: *Though we call upon you in every language / though the birds and trees and oceans speak your name with every breath / there is only one name for you.* And then in "Snowmass" she draws us back to the holy silence with the *song of the invisible One / announcing the now / as only love can do / be still / be still / I am.*

It is through her work as a spiritual teacher in the lineage of Paramahansa Yogananda and as a peace activist that I came to know Ellen Grace O'Brian. I have admired her skill in translating the ancient science of Kriya Yoga in practical, accessible terms for a contemporary audience. I have rejoiced in the well-deserved recognition she has received for contributing to interfaith dialog and pioneering the emerging inter-spiritual movement. I have had the honor of being a guest on her radio show and a speaker at her center, and have been moved by her grounded and humble presence and the deep regard in which her students hold her. But until this glorious collection, *The Moon Reminded Me*, I did not realize what a God-intoxicated ecstatic mystic poet Ellen Grace O'Brian is! In the tradition of my namesake, Mirabai, Ellen knocks on the gates of the heart with her sublime love language and they fly open and the Holy One strides in.

Take your time with these poetic jewels. Breathe them in; breathe them out. The poet engages lyrical language not only to evoke that which transcends all words, but also as a spiritual practice. If we approach the poems in a contemplative way, setting aside the ubiquitous to-do list and making ourselves fully available to the moment, they may become magical portals that allow us to glimpse the face of the Beloved for which our hearts yearn. And if we stay there, we may find ourselves blessed by a direct encounter.

–Mirabai Starr
Taos, New Mexico, February 2017

INTRODUCTION

O Divine Sarasvati, thou art our great destiny,
the ultimate Knowledge,
Divine Beauty with lotus-eyes!
The entire universe is thy form,
thy gaze encircles all the worlds,
Oh Goddess, give us Knowledge!
To You we bow.

My first two books of poetry, *One Heart Opening* and *The Sanctuary of Belonging*, flowed from two streams of my life—one from my experiences as a daughter, wife, mother, and friend; and the other from my experiences as a spiritual pilgrim, a woman of deep longing travelling through India with an open heart. I knew when I wrote this book that those two streams must come together. I knew they belonged together, just as the realm of relationship—the loves and challenges of our earthy life—are inextricably linked to our divine longing and to Self-realization. I wasn't sure how kitchen table metaphors could sit alongside lofty images of temples and divine longing, and still reflect the timeless question: *how do we live our eternal life?* How would these two seemingly disparate streams of body and soul meet and consciously express in the fullness of time?

First, a story. The Sarasvatī River of the Rig Veda, once the site where India's ancient civilization flourished on its banks, has disappeared today. Yet it is envisioned still in hearts and minds as a powerful underground stream. It is said to rise up to meet the two sacred rivers, the Ganges and the Yamuna, at the Triveni Sangam. The Goddess Sarasvatī, whose name means "she of the stream," is the mother of the Vedas, the presiding deity over knowledge and the arts, speech, and writing. According to this legend, when She arrives to join the other two streams, they then triumphantly and gracefully make their way to the sea, the great oneness.

Sit long enough, quietly enough, with the expectation of revelation and it comes. The underground stream of spiritual knowledge and presence began to flow, pervading and connecting the poems in the collection. It was the third stream arising and bringing the necessary confluence of days and eternity. The poems nuanced with Sanskrit gracefully revealed the deeper context to connect the streams. Sanskrit provided the themes of *sandhyā*, transformation; *sankalpa*, intention; *maitrī*, friendship and love; *līlā*, divine play; and ultimately, *Advaita*, the realization of oneness. In most places, the English transliteration of Sanskrit words along with diacritical marks are used with the exception of a few familiar words which have entered the English lexicon, such as Ganges, Rig Veda, or Krishna.

The moon, shining in many of the poems, became the perfect reminder of the divine light reflected in our days and nights, hearts and minds. The arc of the work—from transformation to the realization of oneness—is the prayer of this work and the purview of its poetry. These poems are my humble attempt to put that into words, what I know or suspect but cannot say. I offer them at your lotus feet.

My gratitude for my editor, Parthenia Kavita Hicks, is boundless but not sufficient to honor her inspiration, dedication, direction, and encouragement for this work. For Mirabai Starr, whose life and writing is a light of inspiration to me, I offer profound appreciation for the "yes" to my work and the gift of her brilliant foreword. For L.M. Browning and the team at Homebound Publications who plucked this flower from the field and selected it as finalist in their poetry prize to publish, deep bows of gratitude. For Shanta Bulkin and Indira Bulkin, praṇāms for your profound commitment to Sanskrit and for your generous review of the manuscript. For all of the students, colleagues, and friends who listened as these poems made their way into the heart, I thank you. For my husband, Amarnāth, who unabashedly loves the poems and the poet—I marvel at that divine gift every day. For my guru, Roy Eugene Davis, who made it possible to find the water of the underground stream, eternal gratitude.

–Yogacharya Ellen Grace O'Brian
February 2017

SANDHYĀ
MEETING

SANDHYĀ

Listen.
Lark sings as day begins
and when it ends
the tide of gratitude flows in
senses bow before the One.

This is the hour:
enter the temple of I am That
grace is being dispensed

take *prasād*—ambrosia of now,
nectar of surrender,
it will sweeten your tongue
render you speechless
make you sing.

Sandhyā is Sanskrit for junction and refers to the transitional hours—
the auspicious times of the day for prayer—dawn, noon, and dusk. It
indicates a meeting place, a joining, where two things come together
and become something new.

Prasāda (prasād) is blessed food that is offered to the deity during
worship and then consumed. It also means grace, favor, or a gift
from God.

Rose and Azure Letters

Hari, those rose letters
penned on azure skies
you slipped daily at dawn
under the door

of my mind
called me from my home.
Why hide from me now?
Their fragrance still speaks.

When night jasmine
fills the air
I know: not even
the darkness escapes
your call to bloom.

Hari, which means "the remover" is a Sanskrit name for *Viṣṇu,* also
an epithet of Krishna. It signifies the Lord as the remover of igno-
rance and one's errors.

Īśvara Praṇidhāna

The ocean does not
argue with the rock.
It goes where it will,
telling the secret, again
then again, to the slow
moving cliffs. Prayers
written in moss
answered at dawn.

Listen for the secret.

Be a jagged edge
falling in love
one salty kiss
at a time
see your self
as the shore
longing to dive in
see your self
as the wave
returning home again.

Īśvara Praṇidhāna is Sanskrit for devotion to God, surrendering the
false sense of ego identity, the idea of being separate from the one
Reality.

EVEN THE HUMMINGBIRD

Even the hummingbird stops
at noon to pray
offering the ruby
of praise, the price
of one moment
in the green sanctuary
of belonging.

WINTER

black squirrel green walnut
Zen master in the garden
everything is clear

SHARP EYES

Certain creatures live with
us in the suburbs. Grey squirrels,
mice, and the neon stripped
garden snakes who hunt them.

The neighbor's tiger cat
who could join in
but doesn't, appears
around nine to lap up
rays of sun in the north corner.

Birds—black blue grey yellow
emerge from the side door
of the sky, depart through another
their songs trailing behind them.

At night the party arrives:
no inhibitions raccoon clan,
shy possum family,
power-wielding executive skunks.
Roof rats host it all.

The afternoon he arrived
it took ancient memory
to recognize him. Dog? On
the fence? No. Crimson fur,
sloping tail, triangle face,
sharp eyes.
Fox.

THE MOON REMINDED ME

This morning the moon reminded me
it's never too late, or too early.
Go ahead.

There's a way to turn
without losing your balance
even though you get drunk
on the Beloved's wine
even though you leave
your shoes behind
at the *Sama*. Go ahead
take them off.

Place your hand on your heart
start turning toward the light
raise your self by your Self
at dawn. Go ahead.
Shine in the morning sky.

Sama is a Persian and Arabic word for a ceremony or ritual in the Sufi
tradition that may include music, poetry, prayers, or dancing as a way
of *dhikr*, or divine remembrance. Sufi whirling is a form of *Sama*.

THE TASTE

Winter morning on the coast
sip of steaming coffee
fog clears, sunlight
breaks through tree ferns.

I remember the first taste
of coffee, as a girl
asking, when
will I be old enough?

You said, *whenever you want it
without milk or sugar.*

Black became the real thing,
lifelong love affair
with something bitter
that hints of sweet.

I think of you
your life,
its blows,
your smile.

Oh, I miss you
like a taste
like heat
like bitter
like sweet

Some lessons
from our mothers
arrive years later
with an aftertaste.

HOW WILL I LIVE?

In that ordinary moment
rinsing the dishes
I knew you
had come back

You who were both father and mother
carried our burden into steel mill nights
forging your mind with whiskey's fire
your body covered with black metal ash

Soul rising as foundry flames
burned the dross of desire.

You, who left everyone
including yourself
you came back
free

Stood in the doorway
between the worlds
said to me:
It's true.

I knew your name
was joy then.

What will your visit be
for me? A teacher
revealing love's
power over death?

How will I live?
Now that I know
your real name.

Tides

-i- *Beginnings*

Last year I learned
about small things,
how they determine direction,
set things in motion,
like the trim tab of a great ship.

Day after day, the whales came
so close we could see them,
our eyes naked and astonished.
Rising from the murky depths
mouths open like canyon walls,
the ocean, a river flowing through
skin and teeth, breath shooting up
its salty taste, sky made of sea birds
pelicans, gulls, cormorants, grebes,
flying, diving, swimming,
dolphins and seals at their side.

Think about the anchovy
that brings the whale. The thousands of small acts,
the slippery thoughts, or fast moving words
tumbling from mouth or page, going before us
all the while tugging a line in the universe.

-ii- Endings

One: Mary
We talked on her birthday, laughed, said for six months we would be
the same age, then I would forge ahead again, ever the elder.
This year she said she was tired. She'd been dispensing forgiveness,
making amends with every encounter, told me she forgave me,
said, *You are free* and *I love you.*

You'd have to know Mary
to know that words came easy,
but not those.

Two days later, she was gone.
If you weren't looking or listening,
you might say there was no notice given,
no warning. Yet the goodbyes were shining everywhere,
moving just under the surface of every conversation.

Two: Vivian
Before Vivian left, she wrote notes. Small notes
she posted on things for her daughter to find.
These were your grandmother's pearls.
The key to the safety deposit box is in the bureau.

Inside the safety deposit box, nestled among
the important papers, an envelope marked
open after I am gone. Imagine standing in that vault, alone,
reading: *I have always loved you.* And, *I am so proud of you.*

You'd have to know Vivian
to know that words came easy,
but not those.

Three: Monica
The night that Monica left
the full October moon told me
*No one reflects that much light
without God at the center.*

I wasn't prepared for the news
but if I had really paid attention,
I would have known
Monica was on the move again,
there was no keeping her down.

It's hard to say where
we'll encounter her next—
the song that rises in the heart on a lonely night
and makes you dance in your living room,
that throaty laugh that says
what wisdom can't put into words,
the lights of Paris at night,
sunrise on the coast of Greece,
salty air kissing your face on West Cliff.

I expect her to meet me for dinner at Sabieng,
ride up breathless on her bicycle,
unbuckle her helmet, shake her head,
astound me with her latest revelations, say,
Life is good.

-iii- Remaining

If you want to stay in love
be mindful of the tides,
what they bring in, and take out.
Sharp edges of glass are
smoothed into gems this way.

One day flows into the next
it is all beginning and ending
words becoming flesh
tumbling through time
shining for their moment.

After you have gone, a child will see
green glisten in the sands of time,
pick it up with a small hand,
place it in her pocket,
walk into tomorrow.

Sabieng, a Thai word, means "reserved savory food eaten when some-
one is traveling a great distance."

WORDS

This is how I have left before.
A betrayal, small or large. A stinging word,
a lie, taken in, turned over, folded,
smoothed down, stacked,
methodically placed
one on top of the other
in the suitcase of my mind.

Once full, I closed the lid
fastened the lock
grabbed the handle
walked out the door.

Now I have stopped saving lies
sold my investments
in the currency of shame
watch for the signs
listen when the heart rattles
let my voice sound
feel its weight
stand my ground.

Saṅkalpa

Intention

SAṄKALPA

I was married
to the future.
He made big promises
but never came home.
I tried everything.

Saṅkalpa is a Sanskrit word meaning a wish, volition, or intention.
Its root meaning is "to determine, to come into existence." It is the
mental process we use to assert our will and attempt to control
outcomes.

Hidden Sweetness

I'm looking for some hidden sweetness.
I open a book and read a few words
dust particles in the morning light
swirl in an invisible current
weightless. Not one word sinks
into my heart.

One bite out of every
chocolate in the box.
I'm still searching.

BEFORE DAWN

Before dawn
I walk cool streets
first fires of morning
burn, already
women have touched
their foreheads
with the crimson
of longing

they move
toward you
like brides
their hearts
bouquets
they carry
fragrant
with desire
for you

Swift as birds
they leave
their homes
seek
only you

LATE JANUARY

It is still winter
though we dream
of spring. The branches
of my neighbor's apple tree
reach straight for heaven

rising from winter slumber,
unabashed, wet with grey rain,
no leaf or blossom to adorn them,
no heavy fruit to bend them with humility.

Only this: naked reaching for the light,
so audacious, it stirs the possum in his sleep.

DISCIPLESHIP

Mother
you have shown the doves
where and how to build their nests
in the temple eaves

I am a lost one
the generation
who did not learn to sew
the recipes of my grandmothers
are gone

I left that house.

Now you
must show me
the simple
weaving together
of the soul life.

LISTEN

I am listening
to the sound of your footsteps:
birds coming in to roost
rose petals opening
foam of the wave
disappearing in sand

Women who are asleep
miss the colors of dawn—
the sound of you
coming to meet them.

MUSE

When she visits me
(it is not often, now)
I make a simple offering,
rice from my kitchen
steaming in a small white bowl.
She seasons it, slowly pours
the dark, salty, sauce.

We do not talk, but listen
(to some quieter things)
the movement of clouds,
phantom freight trains
connecting, riding low
across the evening sky.

DESERT MOON

Desert moon rising
wildflowers blooming on sand
what will you do now?

Wings of Red

Sweep the corners
of the heart with a feather,
a breath, a sigh,
a breeze of lovingkindness.

Offer seeds you find
to blackbird
let them be
gold eye flash
red wing promise
dawn flight
from bright grass.

How else to forgive
what we have done?

THE DAY THE MONK SLEPT IN

When I arrived he showed me to my cabin in the woods. "Don't be disturbed if you hear the clinking of glass outside your room in the morning," he said. "It's only me." A few feet from the cabin I could see a small white stucco shrine with niches containing statues of Buddhas facing the four directions, their hands speaking mudras of blessing. On the corners of the shrine were four large bowls filled with water and pink plastic floating flowers. In front of the Buddhas there were many, maybe one hundred and eight, small glass bowls that he filled in the mornings and emptied at dusk, as an offering. "When in the morning?" I asked, "At dawn?" my mind setting the trap to measure the depth of his commitment to prayer. Never mind all this water, I thought. What time do you get up? "Oh no, not at dawn," he smiled. "Maybe around seven or eight." "Oh," I said. I looked at him. He looked American, about thirty-five, a little over-weight, friendly enough, like one of the Conner sons, we grew up with in the suburbs. I found myself glancing at the running shoes peering out from under his maroon and gold robes and somehow his shaved head became a crew cut. I liked him, but at the same time I began to worry, wondering if there was any hope for the world if the forest monks making the offerings to Buddha were now the Conners from next door? In the morning, I woke early and waited at my window. I waited a long time. He did not come. My heart was heavy and my mind was full of judgments. After an hour, it started to rain. It has been raining for four days now. The bowls outside my window overflow.

What is it we know?
Length of days, sunrise, and set.
The grace goes unnoticed.

THE MOON'S DOOR

I have been knocking on the moon's door for hours
she pretends she is not there
but I see slivers of light through the cracks.

Last time she opened the door
I jumped and screamed.
She closed it right away.

What kind of lover
knocks on the door
then screams when you answer?

One who has never before
seen that much beauty.

MAITRĪ

LOVINGKINDNESS

MAITRĪ

It happened like this:
Two geese flew across the sky
their bodies nested in flight
like a married couple familiar
in their bed of years,
their calls a conversation.
Something ancient
woke me to a dream of you.

I thought: you are mine,
as much as I am my own,
which is not at all, yet
we fly together
heading toward home, sometimes
without a thought, just the sky
and the longing that carries us,
allows me to imagine, we.

Maitrī is a Sanskrit word meaning friendship, love, benevolence, or
lovingkindness.

Fire in my Heart

Some days I sit near your fire
feeding it the kindling of desire.
Live in the way, the Buddha said,
and the light will grow in you.

Sorrow and joy come in
sit down together as friends.
Everything that is needed appears.

Other days I forget about the light
set out alone in the dark—
ambitious prodigal with damp wood
determined to start my own fire.

When the invitation to the heavenly feast
arrives from the universe, I politely decline.
I have prepared a feast for you,
will you come?

No, I am too busy
with matters of life and death.
I insist on my own way, saying no to love
until no becomes sand in my mouth.
Why all this suffering I ask?

Come, sit by the fire,
forget about life and death
being and doing
coming and going.

Soon the sitar will begin,
its notes will make you weep
for everything lost and gained
for the extravagant mercy of the One.

SEEING MY FATHER AT LAST

Cancer broke the locks
on your heart, burned
through the hinges
of your control.

Words burst into flame
leapt from your mouth
like wild horses in a fire
that frightened even you.

Listen to me! you said
Why did I say that?

You shake your head in disbelief,
the wild horse drinks from the stream,
grazes in an open meadow.

You say: *If I keep on like this
everyone will be gone.*

Light comes through
the window, I notice
the quiver of your chin
feel my heart open.

Salt for the Bread

There are times when
you are cut, and I
move toward you
with water for the wound.
But the heat of anger
between us
turns it to salt.

Who does this?
A man, a good man,
and a woman,
a good woman.
They love each other
but for a brief time,
flirt with pride.

Salt sits on the table
next to the sweet bread.

Now We Learn about Love

The springbox doesn't consider
whether or not to overflow
whether or not to pour herself forth

free from calculating
how much or not enough
every moment
she gives herself away
yet every moment
she is full.

If you ask her
how she does this
she falls over laughing

The Mother's Compassion

Dawn slid silently
through trees this morning
gently waking sparrows
in their nests

As she pulled back
the blanket of fog
she whispered, *Joy is near—*
Wake up, Wake up

A Dove Year

A pomegranate year

ripe and cracked open
rubies pour forth inspiration
staining our days with curious hope

A dove year

white lace of its tail
at home on the ground or in the air
soft cries caress the hearts of lovers
leaving their windows open to morning

A year of children

leafy green and flowering wild
gather wounded saints from the field
bringing them in the house of courage
where they live on and on

everyone has a place at this table
innocence and experience sit side by side
weaving conversations with strands of time

Gandhi and Rumi discuss
the merits of spinning
and Martin says to Bobby, *Look,*
the dream goes on.

WHERE ANGELS KEEP THE GREEN

Blake has been walking
in my garden at night
mumbling under his breath
rose, oh rose
peering under the last
leaves of winter
rose, oh rose

My daughter, my father,
and some of my friends, join him.
He shows them the winter garden
stalks adorned with thorns
says *if you look close enough*
the red of next year's rose
shows itself in the wood.

I ask him about the angels
He says this: *the first*
half of life is gathering;
sing a song of innocence.
The second is letting go;
experience brings its own song.

The angels tend the garden.
If you want to know
the One who sent them
keep your heart open.

There is nothing
for you to do, only this—
keep your heart open—
it is the red in the wood
this winter's day.

On a dry branch
hummingbird sings
rose, oh rose

AMARNĀTH

I
Flowers in the garden—
wild iris, abutilon,
white heritage rose—
refuse to come inside,
sit in a vase,
grace my table.

A moment ago
singing in the earth,
dancing in the sun,
they drop limp in my arms—
nonviolent resisters,
who won't cooperate.

The words I look for
to say I love you
cannot be spoken—
the blessing of being is
whispered and shouted
by every common thing.

II
The water lily rests
upon the lake
and opens.

The heart makes
the body radiant.
Radha lives only for Krishna.
And me? I am
because of you.
Can you imagine me
without you?
Impossible!

Amarnāth is a Sanskrit name meaning Immortal Lord. It is another
name for *Lord Śiva* (Shiva), Supreme Reality. *Rādhā* (Radha) and
Kṛṣṇa (Krishna) the eternal couple, can represent the love of the soul
and Spirit.

TO THE GURU OF THE PASSING YEAR

To the Guru of the passing year
I bow, and say *Namaste!*
I behold the divine in you
I pause, and say *thank you*
for every teaching

though I'm a poor student
don't finish my assignments
want credit for it all
yearn for recess
fall asleep during class

need a bell to wake up
yet love learning as light
loves the empty room
at the end of the day

thank you
for the teachings that woke me
and for those I slept through

I walk out with the nod of your blessing
as the door of this year closes behind me.

Guru is a Sanskrit word meaning teacher, the light that removes the darkness of ignorance. The term can apply to one's teacher; to God, the Teacher of all teachers; or to Life itself with its inherent tendency to support spiritual awakening and the fulfillment of its purposes.

LĪLĀ

Divine Play

LĪLĀ

Your *līlā*
 is impossible.

In your *līlā*
winning comes only
through surrender.
What kind of victory is that?

Līlā is a Sanskrit word meaning divine play. It is the cosmic play, the
idea that creation itself exists for the pure joy of it.

RADIANCE

This is how radiance
breaks out

those afraid to sing
find their voices
shopkeepers lose count
and begin to dance

the underground stream
leaps into the ocean
the darkest night
provokes the day

the teacher weeps
the infant speaks
all debts are forgotten

Any moment becomes new
in me, and in you,
when radiance
breaks out

A LOVER'S QUESTION

Trying to walk a simple path with cleverness
is like trying to answer your lover's question
by looking in a book.

Do you love me? I don't know
let me look it up.

CROWS

The crows are flying around the neighborhood
cooking up a wild day. One says: *Come on!*
And his slick black-winged buddies follow.

Later I see them nipping at the heels
of the local vulture, sending her into a tailspin.
It's a day too mischievous for death.

I think the poem ends here.

From the tallest branch they cry:
Haw, haw. Haw, haw.

INDRIYAS

My five girlfriends
are after you.
One has gone shopping
for something to catch your eye—
a tight skirt, short, and
high heels with an ankle strap.
She thinks the legs may do it.

Her friend is working late
preparing papers for you
convinced that when the last
one is finished and filed
you will arrive to congratulate her.

The others have their own ways as well.
One looks for you in the veteran's hospital
among young men wounded in the war
while her friend stays home and prays
offering mantras and incense for the sick and dying.

Another one cleans the house
arranges flowers on the table
shops for organic food.
She looks for you in the market
imagines you sitting at her table
at last captured by grace and beauty.

I know they're all foolish women
yet sometimes I get so lonely for you
I join them and play along.

Indriyas, Sanskrit for sense organs, refers to our instruments of
expression and perception, which include our five sense abilities to
see, hear, smell, taste, and touch. The senses are considered unreliable
avenues to divine knowledge, which transcends sensory perception.

Svadharma

I've become obsessed with prayer
I wonder: are the frogs
saying *Allah! Allah!* Or
Rama, Rama, Rama?
Perhaps it's *Jesus! Jesus!*
My Buddhist friend says
I have it all wrong.
He's certain they are saying
Froggy! Froggy!
Everyone has their own song.

Svadharma is Sanskrit for one's own true path, way, duty, or natural expression.

I CANNOT USE WHAT
YOU HAVE GIVEN ME

I cannot use
what you have given me
when I try to give it away
it returns.

They do not want it
in the marketplace, there
flower vendors tie
white jasmine together
for other women's hair.

I am uncovered
unadorned
wear
only
that

I HAVE NOT TOLD OTHER WOMEN

I have not told
the other women
how you met me
in that secret place
and made the honey drip.

So many of them tell
lies about you,
your name rolls
off their tongues.

Before we met I could
talk with them, now
I am mute
after meeting you
everything I say
is a betrayal.

LARK SINGING
THROUGH THE NIGHT

I've given up the ledger,
remain hopelessly in debt.
Every time I say *thank you*
a new gift appears at my door.

Your love has cured me
of the madness that imagines
I am generous.

Now I know
I am a spring overflowing
a lark singing through the night
and yes, the full moon shining,
a brilliant borrowed light.

The moon was so full tonight

The moon was so
full tonight
the waves
rolled over laughing.
They're in cahoots.

As soon as the sky
runs out of blue
the waves call
the moon over and
raise up their skirts
for a wild night.

After they quiet down
a glistening white stripe
appears on the wet sand.

Listen: after the tide slips out
a drunken chorus arises.
When everything is spent
a love song remains.
They are singing
a sweet song about you.
They all love you.

Like the rest of us
they'd do anything
to bring your radiance
a little closer.

SATSANGA

In late afternoon
wind and redwoods
get together to talk
about the ocean.

They are remembering
mist that arrived before dawn:
call it manna,
or grace.

The trees make a vow
to stand all night
so they won't miss it.

Satsaṅga (satsang) is Sanskrit for a gathering of devotees. It refers to
being in holy company, those who come together for spiritual study
and remembrance, especially in the presence of a guru.

MANTRA

To keep his donkey close
the merchant ties
its front legs together.
Now it cannot wander
this donkey can be trusted
near his neighbor's carrots.
The merchant is free to work
all day without worry.

At dusk, he unties this
tendency to wander, and
together, they go home.

I tie the mischief of my mind
with the rope of your name.
It's dusk and I'm waiting
for you. Untie the knot.
Let's go home.

Mantra is a Sanskrit word indicating particular sacred words or
phrases that aid in transcending the thinking mind, or thought
activity. As a tool for meditation, mantra is used to focus attention
and clear the mind of distraction, making the experience of divine
union possible.

ADVAITA
ONENESS

PLAYING ADVAITA WITH GOD

In the great marble game
I told God I wanted
His big cat's eye shooter.
Ok, He said,
You can have the cat's eye,
if you give Me all your marbles.
The deal was at hand.
The moment: now.

No time to think of holding back—
pure crystals, aggies, or blue sky pearls.
Ok! I said, emptying out my bag,
feeling the rush of the exchange,
thinking: what a bargain!
When you play with God,
you can lose all your marbles
and still be smiling.

Just as my mind began to sing:
I've won! I've won!
My heart noticed
the game was over.
One marble can't take anyone out,
its circle is everywhere.

Just about the time I begin to get it,
God opens His blue velvet pouch
and returns all the marbles.
The circle is already full,
but every day He sends more.
The line between in and out has disappeared.
What kind of a game is this?

Grab the cat's eye shooter
let's play!

Advaita is the Vedanta philosophy of the great oneness of all that is.
The term means nonduality, or literally, "not-two."

THE KEY

What use is ritual
to the One?
Why look for the key
when you're inside the shop?
In that moment, who can buy?
Who can sell? Why browse for the jewels
sewn inside your own coat?

Hummingbird says:
The red jewel stays hidden
without a song.
When the throat opens
to sing of the One,
the ruby appears.

One Name

Though we call upon you
in every language
though the birds and trees
and oceans speak your name
with every breath, there is only
one name for you—

it resounds in every sigh
in the breath of lovers
cry of the newborn
rattle of the dying
and the silence
that remains

spoken by every tongue
both eloquent and mute
it gathers us
in your wild embrace.

I am tempted to say
your name is Love
but it is not.

Or perhaps it is.

I cannot say your name
yet I know: it sings in our blood
sounding through the universe
whirling in the bright night.

OM

Which comes first?
ocean or rain?
fire or wood?
scent of water
or trees bursting into bloom?
lover who is lost
or Beloved who finds?

You are the ocean
drinking in the rain
that you, yourself, have made.

You are the fire in the wood.
You are the scent of water
and the trees bursting into bloom.

Fire lives in water, as darkness
lives in everything green, as time
slips out of eternity.

A luminous thread connects
lover and Beloved
prayer beads travel on it
chanting the Name Om,
Om that is everything.

Om, is Sanskrit for the Word, the Eternal, the divine power that brings everything into expression. All words, all creation, are considered to be various forms of this one sound. It is the great divine Name.

ANĀHATA

Listen with presence
like the fingers of a cellist
listen to the strings

Like the moon listens to the sun
like a bee listens to the fuchsia bell
and loses himself in the whorl

Like the mind listens to the heart
tastes the sound of bliss
and meets the Self again.

Anāhata is a Sanskrit term for the heart chakra, or heart center. It means "unstruck." As anāhata-nada it refers to the Om vibration, the holy Word, the eternal resonance of the divine presence in everyone and everything.

SNOWMASS

I spent the afternoon in heaven
brought a book along
(bare necessity).
Ah, serenity.

Even heaven is not quiet.
The aspens were singing
psalms from Mt. Sopris
thousand tongued chorus
green upon green delight
song of the invisible One
announcing the now
as only love can do
be still, be still
I Am.

In the heart is a well

In the heart
is a well, filled
with the sound
of silence.
Drink

from it.
One
taste
changes
everything.

How do I know?
The day I stopped
sitting on the edge
and fell in,
told me this.

The Beloved's Gift

Everything shines in the pure light of morning.

We, even we, who close our eyes at night
weary of the world, awaken each day
the glimmering kiss of the Beloved
still shining upon our brows

The call comes.

Blades of grass hear it
standing in the meadow as brides
wearing beads of radiance
the color of surrender

Hear the call.

Hasten to prayer
as they do, turn to the One
who has kissed you
bend before love

WAKING

A prayer
rises in my chest at dawn
sounds its way
through my throat
into the day
joins the chorus of finches
outside the open window

The time for gratitude is early
long before the train
of forgetfulness
arrives.

MĀYĀ

Buddha points to the earth
Zen master points to the moon
Arjuna points to the target
Mary points to her child
Jesus points to the heart
Rumi points to Shams

We all look
until we see

Māyā is Sanskrit for illusion, the principle of appearance, the power
and mystery of creation, that which conceals our divine nature. It
allows the Absolute, which is free from attributes, to express as
having qualities.

Shams-i-Tabrīzī was Jalāl ad-Dīn Muhammad Rūmī's spiritual
teacher, friend, or shaykh.

TOUCH THE EARTH

Leave this place
in the fall
like
a
leaf

like the Buddha
touch the earth
witness
let
go

SOMEONE HAS LEFT
THE DOOR OPEN

Fantastic!
Someone has left the door open to the inner sanctum.
Now all the pilgrims are running back home
shouting praises, their faces radiant
with the light that surrender brings.

Turn around and you'll see—
the One you've been looking for
has found you.

ABOUT THE AUTHOR

Yogacharya Ellen Grace O'Brian, M.A., poet, writer, and teacher is founder and spiritual director of the Center for Spiritual Enlightenment (CSE), a meditation center in the ancient tradition of Kriya Yoga (www.CSEcenter.org). She was ordained to teach in 1982 by Roy Eugene Davis, a direct disciple of Paramahansa Yogananda. She teaches throughout the US and internationally and is the recipient of the Hindu American Foundation's 2015 Mahatma Gandhi Award for the advancement of religious pluralism. She is vice chair emeritus of the Parliament of the World's Religions and president of the Board of Carry the Vision, a nonprofit organization for nonviolence education. Her books include *Living the Eternal Way: Spiritual Meaning and Practice in Daily Life* and *A Single Blade of Grass: Finding the Sacred in Everyday Life*. She is the founding editor of *Enlightenment Journal*, a quarterly yoga magazine; a regular contributor to *Truth Journal* magazine; and *Contemplative Journal* online; as well as host of *The Yoga Hour*, a weekly radio program that brings contemporary writers and spiritual leaders together in conversation about yoga, world religions, and spirituality. She is the author of two previous volumes of poetry—*One Heart Opening* and *The Sanctuary of Belonging*, published by CSE Press. Her work is included in the anthology, *Poetic Medicine*, by John Fox. As a western meditation teacher, poet, and writer, Yogacharya O'Brian weaves poetry throughout her teachings as a way to communicate what words can only point to. Her work exemplifies the universal nature of yoga philosophy and makes its wisdom accessible to people from all walks of life.

WWW.ELLENGRACEOBRIAN.COM

Acknowledgments

I'm grateful to John Fox for including my poem, "Muse," in *Poetic Medicine/The Healing Art of Poem-Making*, Penguin Putnam Publishers.

"Mother" appeared in *Living the Eternal Way/Spiritual Meaning and Practice in Daily Life* published by CSE Press and in the present manuscript as "Discipleship."

The following poems appeared in *The Sanctuary of Belonging*, CSE Press, and are included in the present manuscript, most of them with revisions:

"Even the Hummingbird"
"Before Dawn (Before dawn I walk)"
"Listen (I've been listening)"
"Rose and Azure Letters (Hari, those rose letters)"
"Discipleship (Mother)"
"In the heart is a well"
"I cannot use what you have given me"
"I have not told the other women"

The following poems appeared in *One Heart Opening: Poems for the Journey of Awakening*, CSE Press, and are included in the present manuscript, most of them with revisions:

"Muse"
"Īśvara Praṇidhāna"
"The Day the Monk Slept In"

HOMEBOUND PUBLICATIONS

Ensuring that the mainstream isn't the only stream.

At Homebound Publications, we publish books written by independent voices for independent minds. Our books focus on a return to simplicity and balance, connection to the earth and each other, and the search for meaning and authenticity. Founded in 2011, Homebound Publications is one of the rising independent publishers in the country. Collectively through our imprints, we publish between fifteen to twenty offerings each year. Our authors have received dozens of awards, including: *Foreword Reviews'* Book of the Year, Nautilus Book Award, Benjamin Franklin Book Awards, and Saltire Literary Awards. Highly-respected among bookstores, readers and authors alike, Homebound Publications has a proven devotion to quality, originality and integrity.

We are a small press with big ideas. As an independent publisher we strive to ensure that the mainstream is not the only stream. It is our intention at Homebound Publications to preserve contemplative storytelling. We publish full-length introspective works of creative non-fiction as well as essay collections, travel writing, poetry, and novels. In all our titles, our intention is to introduce new perspectives that will directly aid humankind in the trials we face at present as a global village.

WWW.HOMEBOUNDPUBLICATIONS.COM

CPSIA information can be obtained
at www.ICGtesting.com
Printed in the USA
FSOW01n0344221216
28558FS